Freedom From Acne

Dr. Robert B. Campbell Th.D.

Pool of Bethesda

4647 Reservoir Rd., Geneseo, NY 14454
www.poolofbethesda.org

poolofbethesdaschoolofhealing@gmail.com

ISBN-13: 978-1494781248

ISBN-10: 1494781247

DEDICATION

This book is dedicated to all those who have been afflicted with Acne. May you find freedom as you read about the process that has brought others their freedom.

DISCLAIMER

We are not in competition with nor do not seek to be in conflict with any medical or psychiatric practices, counseling, etc. We do not practice medicine nor do we practice psychology. We are not responsible for anyone's disease or healing. We share insights. All of our work is intended to give insights into healing as we look at possible spiritual roots to disease, sickness and infirmity. We cannot and do not guarantee healing. We have seen incredible results in our work with others. Our insights are not meant to substitute for medical advice or treatment. We do not diagnose or treat disease. We encourage you to seek medical care for your health issues.

All Scriptures are quoted from The New King James Version of the Bible unless stated otherwise.

ACKNOWLEDGMENTS

There are so many that I have drawn from over the years in my search to find healing and wholeness not only for myself but others. My greatest insights have come from my time in the Word of God. Jesus I am thankful!

Isaiah 35:3-10 **Energize** *the limp hands,* **strengthen** *the rubbery knees. 4* **Tell fearful souls***, "Courage! Take heart! God is here, right here, on his way to put things right And redress all wrongs. He's on his way! He'll save you!" 5* **Blind eyes** *will be opened,* **deaf ears** *unstopped, 6* **Lame men and women** *will leap like deer,* **the voiceless** *break into song.* **Springs of water will burst out in the wilderness, streams flow in the desert***. 7* **Hot sands will become a cool oasis, thirsty ground a splashing fountain***. Even lowly jackals will have* **water to drink, and barren grasslands flourish richly***. 8 There will be a highway called the Holy Road. No one rude or rebellious is permitted on this road. It's for God's people exclusively —impossible to get lost on this road. Not even fools can get lost on it. 9 No lions on this road, no dangerous wild animals — Nothing and no one dangerous or threatening. Only the redeemed will walk on it. 10 The people God has ransomed will come back on this road.* **They'll sing as they make their way home to Zion, unfading halos of joy encircling their heads, Welcomed home with gifts of joy and gladness as all sorrows and sighs scurry into the night.** *MSG*

INTRODUCTION

I want to share with you what I would say to you if I were speaking to you face to face about acne. These insights and principles have helped bring healing to many people over the years through one on one ministry or in our healing schools. I pray these insights will bring healing and release from acne. These principles are not intended to be head knowledge applied only once, but to be revelation, walked out all through life. If you just try this, it will have limited impact, but if you get the full revelation, you will walk in a changed mindset until you see the full manifestation of your healing!

Table of Contents

Chapter 1
Acne

Acne

Most kids get acne at one time or another. The ratio is about 8 in 10 who get acne as a teen or pre- teen. There are approximately 17 million people in the United States who have acne. That's a lot of acne sufferers! Of course being aware that you are not alone does not solve the problem. So what is acne?

Acne is a skin condition that shows up as different types of bumps. They include whiteheads, blackheads, red bumps (pimples), and bumps that are filled with pus (pustules). What causes these annoying bumps? Well, your skin is covered with tiny holes called hair follicles, or pores. Pores contain sebaceous (say: suh-bay-shus) glands (also called oil glands) that make sebum (say: see-bum), an oil that moistens your hair and skin.

Most of the time the glands make the right amount of sebum, and the pores are fine. But sometimes a pore gets clogged up with too much sebum, dead skin cells, and germs called bacteria. This can cause acne.

*If a pore gets clogged up, closes, and bulges out from the skin, that's a **whitehead**. If a pore clogs up but stays open, the top surface can get dark and you're left with a **blackhead**. Sometimes the walls of the pore are broken, allowing sebum, bacteria, and dead skin cells to get under the skin. This causes a small, red infection called* *a pimple. Clogged-up pores that open up deep in the skin can lead to bigger infections known as cysts.*[1]

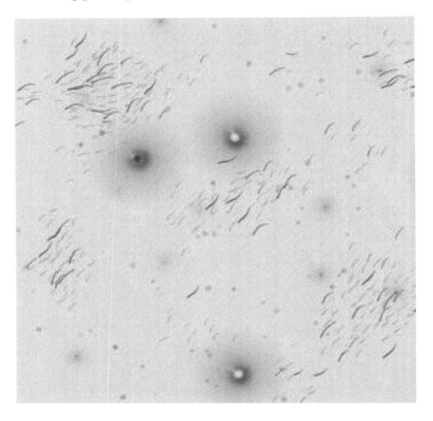

What Causes Acne?

By Mayo Clinic Staff[2]

Three factors contribute to the formation of acne:

- *Overproduction of oil (sebum)*
- *Irregular shedding of dead skin cells resulting in irritation of the hair follicles of your skin*

---

[1] http://kidshealth.org/kid/grow/body_stuff/acne.html#

[2] http://www.mayoclinic.org/diseases-conditions/acne/basics/causes/con-20020580

- *Buildup of bacteria*

Acne occurs when the hair follicles become plugged with oil and dead skin cells. Hair follicles are connected to sebaceous glands. These glands secrete an oily substance known as sebum to lubricate your hair and skin. Sebum normally travels up along the hair shafts and then out through the openings of the hair follicles onto the surface of your skin. When your body produces an excess amount of sebum and dead skin cells, the two can build up in the hair follicles and form together as a soft plug, creating an environment where bacteria can thrive.

This plug may cause the follicle wall to bulge and produce a whitehead. Or, the plug may be open to the surface and may darken, causing a blackhead. Pimples are raised red spots with a white center that develop when blocked hair follicles become inflamed or infected. Blockages and inflammation that develop deep inside hair follicles produce lumps beneath the surface of your skin called cysts. Other pores in your skin, which are the openings of the sweat glands onto your skin, aren't normally involved in acne.

Factors that may worsen acne

These factors can trigger or aggravate an existing case of acne:

- **Hormones.** *Androgens are hormones that increase in boys and girls during puberty and cause the sebaceous glands to enlarge and make more sebum. Hormonal* *changes related to pregnancy and the use of oral contraceptives can also affect sebum production.*

- **Certain medications.** *Drugs containing corticosteroids, androgens or lithium are known to cause acne.*
- **Diet.** *Studies indicate that certain dietary factors, including dairy products and carbohydrate-rich foods — such as bread, bagels and chips, which increase blood sugar — may trigger acne.*

Acne myths

Contrary to what some people think, these factors have little effect on acne:

- **Greasy foods and chocolate** *have proved to have little to no effect on the development or course of acne.*
- **Dirty skin.** *Acne isn't caused by dirt. In fact, scrubbing the skin too hard or cleansing with harsh soaps or chemicals irritates the skin and can make acne worse. Simple cleansing of the skin to remove excess oil and dead skin cells is all that's required.*

Here are a couple of interesting factors to consider when examining what causes acne. It can be **hereditary**. In other words, if your parents had it, you are prone to get it as well. Another factor that can contribute to acne is **stress**. When you feel stressed your pores will make more sebum. Of course you can also suffer with **emotional distress** as a result of having acne as well. We will look into how to deal with these three factors in particular, later in the book. On a positive note, most people outgrow acne by the time they reach their twenties.

Stress and Acne from Acne.org

The mind and the body are connected. This is not Eastern philosophy, it is undisputable physical reality. Emotional stress affects our endocrine (hormone) system, digestive system, respiratory system, immune system, and various other bodily systems. We know that stress can aggravate acne, but exactly why remains a mystery.[3]

Q *Are stress and acne related?*

A *Yes. Stress can aggravate symptoms, but we can almost always overcome* the acne produced as a result of moderate or light stress with proper topical treatment.

Q *What exactly is "stress" anyway?*

A *Stress is any taxing of our emotional or physical being. Widely defined this can include pretty much everything, but for our purposes we'll define it as any undue emotional or physical strain. It might be surprising that this definition includes physical strain. Many people view stress as just an emotional issue, but when we're speaking about acne, it is best to include undue physical strain in our definition since both can come into play.*

Examples of emotional stress:

- *Anxiety regarding an upcoming big event, like a wedding or important test*
- *Bullying*
- *Relationship problems*
- *Overwhelming workload*
- *Health of a loved one*

---

[3] http://www.acne.org/causes-of-acne.html

Examples of physical stress:

- *Overly demanding sports or exercise schedule without adequate rest*
- *Lack of sleep*
- *A hectic lifestyle which can lead to physical tension and shallow breathing*
- *A sedentary lifestyle*
- *Smoking/Drugs*

Q How does stress affect acne?

A The average acne sufferer's skin contains clogged pores that they can't even see. Stress causes an inflammatory response in the body and can cause the walls of these pores to break. When this happens, the body responds with redness around the broken pore, and an influx of pus (a zit).

Also, when we experience stress, our adrenal gland goes into overdrive. Androgens (male hormones), which this gland produces, increase. Higher androgen levels can lead to more acne. This is especially true in women, who produce a much larger percentage of their androgens in the adrenal gland than men. This may explain why stress seems to affect women more than men when it comes to acne.[4]

It is also interesting that acne in women is a growing problem. I believe one reason for this is that there are many more women in the workplace than ever before. They are also in positions of leadership that produce stressful environments to work in. This is not meant to be a sexist statement, but rather an observation of the increased stress in women's lives as a result of the change in the culture. When you are in a place of increased responsibility, stress

---

[4] http://www.acne.org/stress-and-acne.html

increases and women naturally produce a larger percentage of androgens in the adrenal gland than men. Stress and stress related illnesses are on the rise as well.[5]

From the Mayo Clinic

Factors that may worsen acne
These factors can trigger or aggravate an existing case of acne:

Hormones. *Androgens are hormones that increase in boys and girls during puberty and cause the sebaceous glands to enlarge and make more sebum. Hormonal changes related to pregnancy and the use of oral contraceptives can also affect sebum production.*

(Hormones likely play a role in the development of adult acne, but hormones generally aren't the root cause of acne.

It's true that some people with hormonal imbalances due to diseases such as polycystic ovary syndrome experience more problems with acne. However, the vast majority of those with adult acne have no measurable hormonal imbalance.

A number of so-called natural acne treatments promise to "equalize" hormonal imbalances to reduce adult acne breakouts. But "natural hormones" are often derived from plants. Their chemical structure is different from hormones produced in the body, so their effectiveness may be

---

[5] http://www.theguardian.com/business/2011/oct/05/stress-commonest-cause-long-term-sick-leave

limited. And because hormonal imbalance isn't thought to play a major role in acne anyway, the premise behind such products is shaky at best.)[6]

Certain medications. *Drugs containing corticosteroids, androgens or lithium are known to cause acne.*

Diet. *Studies indicate that certain dietary factors, including dairy products and carbohydrate-rich foods — such as bread, bagels and chips, which increase blood sugar — may trigger acne.*

Acne myths
Contrary to what some people think, these factors have little effect on acne:

Greasy foods and chocolate *have proved to have little to no effect on the development or course of acne.*

Dirty skin. *Acne isn't caused by dirt. In fact, scrubbing the skin too hard or cleansing with harsh soaps or chemicals irritates the skin and can make acne worse. Simple cleansing of the skin to remove excess oil and dead skin cells is all that's required.*[7]

Acne: Tips for managing

You can reduce your acne by following these skin care tips from dermatologists.

---

[6] http://www.mayoclinic.org/diseases-conditions/acne/expert-answers/adult-acne/FAQ-20058129
[7] http://www.mayoclinic.com/health/acne/DS00169/DSECTION=causes

1. *Wash twice a day and after sweating. Perspiration, especially when wearing a hat or helmet, can make acne worse, so wash your skin as soon as possible after sweating.*

2. *Use your fingertips to apply a gentle, non-abrasive cleanser. Using a washcloth, mesh sponge or anything else can irritate the skin.*

3. *Be gentle with your skin. Use gentle products, such as those that are alcohol-free. Do not use products that irritate your skin, which may include astringents, toners and exfoliants. Dry, red skin makes acne appear worse.*

4. *Scrubbing your skin can make acne worse. Avoid the temptation to scrub your skin.*

5. *Rinse with lukewarm water.*

6. *Shampoo regularly. If you have oily hair, shampoo daily.*

7. *Let your skin heal naturally. If you pick, pop or squeeze your acne, your skin will take longer to clear and you increase the risk of getting acne scars.*

8. *Keep your hands off your face. Touching your skin throughout the day can cause flare-ups.*

9. *Stay out of the sun and tanning beds. Tanning damages you skin. In addition, some acne medications make the skin very sensitive to ultraviolet (UV) light, which you get from both the sun and indoor tanning devices.*

   - *Using tanning beds increases your risk for melanoma, the deadliest form of skin cancer, by 75 percent.*

10. Consult a dermatologist if:

- *Your acne makes you shy or embarrassed.*

- *The products you've tried have not worked.*

- *Your acne is leaving scars or darkening your skin.*

Today, virtually every case of acne can be successfully treated. Dermatologists can help treat existing acne, prevent new breakouts and reduce your chance of developing scars. If you have questions or concerns about caring for your skin, you should make an appointment to see a dermatologist.[8]

---

[8] http://www.aad.org/dermatology-a-to-z/diseases-and-treatments/a---d/acne/tips

Chapter 2
Disease, Illness and the Immune System

Your body needs to neutralize and get rid of waste materials produced during metabolism. When the immune system weakens, the body finds itself unable to fight toxic substances alone. This raises the levels of toxins and ultimately, the inner detoxification system gets weak, and you have more (acne) breakouts.[9]

Because so many diseases and illnesses are tied to the health of the immune system, I feel it important that we understand how the immune system works, or, in many cases, doesn't work.

About the Immune System

The immune system protects the body against infectious invaders such as germs, viruses, bacteria and even cancer cells. It is like the police force of your body arresting the bad guys and getting rid of them. This police force is comprised of special cells, organs and tissues that all work cooperatively to protect you. Did you know that even bacteria, which is so small that more than a million could fit on the head of a pin, have systems that protect them against infection by viruses?[10]

---

[9] http://www.webmd.com/skin-problems-and-treatments/acne/acne-care-11/lifestyle
[10] http://www.historyofvaccines.org/content/articles/human-immune-system-and-infectious-disease

A major part of the immune system is the lymphatic system which is comprised of a network of vessels and lymph nodes. The lymph nodes are small bean shaped structures that produce and store cells that fight infection and disease. The vessels of the lymph nodes are thin tubes that branch out into all the tissues of the body much like blood vessels. These tubes carry a liquid called lymph that contains tissue fluid, waste products, and immune system cells (white blood cells or leukocytes). It is the white blood cells that trap viruses, bacteria, other invaders and even cancer cells. The white blood cells are made in one of the lymph organs, the bone marrow. [11] Organs and tissues involved in the immune system include bone marrow, lymph nodes, appendix, tonsils, spleen and the thymus.[12] When the body is fighting infection the lymph nodes can become sore and swollen.

Two Types of Leukocytes

Leukocytes are produced or stored in many locations in the body, including the thymus, spleen, and bone marrow. For this reason, they're called the lymphoid organs. There are also clumps of lymphoid tissue throughout the body, primarily as lymph nodes, that house the leukocytes.

The leukocytes circulate through the body between the organs and nodes via lymphatic vessels and

---

[11] Adapted from
http://www.urmc.rochester.edu/Encyclopedia/Content.aspx?ContentTypeID=134&ContentID=123
[12] http://www.historyofvaccines.org/content/articles/human-immune-system-and-infectious-disease

blood vessels. In this way, the immune system works in a coordinated manner to monitor the body for germs or substances that might cause problems.

The two basic types of leukocytes are:

1. **phagocytes**, cells that chew up invading organisms.

2. **lymphocytes**, cells that allow the body to remember and recognize previous invaders and help the body destroy them.

A number of different cells are considered phagocytes. The most common type is the **neutrophil**, which primarily fights bacteria. If doctors are worried about a bacterial infection, they might order a blood test to see if a patient has an increased number of neutrophils triggered by the infection. Other types of phagocytes have their own jobs to make sure that the body responds appropriately to a specific type of invader.

The two kinds of lymphocytes are **B lymphocytes** and **T lymphocytes**. Lymphocytes start out in the bone marrow and either stay there and mature into B cells, or they leave for the thymus gland, where they mature into T cells. B lymphocytes and T lymphocytes have separate functions: B lymphocytes are like the body's military intelligence system, seeking out their targets and sending defenses to lock onto them. T cells are like *the soldiers, destroying the invaders that the intelligence system has identified.[13]*

How a Healthy Immune System Works

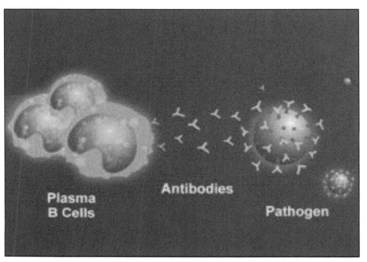

Infection occurs when invaders enter the body cells and reproduce. Viruses, bacteria, and parasites have proteins on their outer surfaces, that are not normally found in the human body. Your immune system sees these foreign substances as antigens. When antigens (invaders) enter the body and are detected, several cell types recognize them and respond to the threat. This is what happens when we get a cold or flu. These cells alert the B lymphocytes (B cells) to produce antibodies that will lock onto the invaders much like attaching a flag. Once these antibodies are produced, they continue to exist in our bodies, so that if those same invaders come into the body again, those

---

[13] http://kidshealth.org/parent/general/body_basics/immune.html

antibodies are ready to do their job again, identifying the invaders. *Image source¹⁴*

The antibodies can identify and lock onto the invaders, but they are unable to destroy the invader without the help of the T lymphocytes or T cells. The T cells (killer cells), are designed to destroy the antigens that are flagged by the B cells. The T cells actually bump up against the invaders and kill them. T cells also help signal other cells to do their job, or once the threat is contained, when to stop the attack. This is why when a person gets a disease like chickenpox, they do not usually get it again, as the antibodies remain in the system.¹⁵

What Can Go Wrong?

Basically there are 3 potential immune system disorders. You can have either a weak or underactive immune system, an overactive immune system, or an immune system that turns against you called an autoimmune disease.

Examples of diseases related to an underactive immune system would include but not be limited to SCID or "bubble boy disease", and AIDS.

Examples of diseases related to an overactive immune system would include but not be limited to Asthma (see my book Freedom From Asthma)¹⁶, Allergies, Eczema (see my

---

[14] http://www.historyofvaccines.org/content/articles/human-immune-system-and-infectious-disease
[15] Adapted from http://kidshealth.org/parent/general/body_basics/immune.html
[16] http://www.amazon.com/Freedom-Asthma-Pool-Bethesda-3/dp/1493700758/ref=la_B00DRGNZLU_1_6?s=books&ie=UTF8&qid=1387841102&sr=1-6

book Freedom From Eczema)[17] and Acne. An overactive immune system is typically responding to stressors.

Examples of diseases related to an autoimmune system disorder would include but not be limited to Type 1 diabetes, Rheumatoid Arthritis, and Lupus.[18]

Cancers of the Immune System

Cancer occurs when cells grow out of control. This also can happen with the cells of the immune system. Leukemia, which involves abnormal overgrowth of leukocytes, is the most common childhood cancer. Lymphoma involves the lymphoid tissues and is one of the more common childhood cancers. With current medications most cases of both types of cancer in kids and teens are curable.[19]

What Are Some Causes of Immune System Imbalance?

Some of the major contributors to problems in the immune system are our emotions such as anger, fear, bitterness and stress. Researchers have scientifically linked emotions to heart disease, high blood pressure, and diseases related to the immune system. Studies have also shown the correlation of emotions to allergies, infections and autoimmune diseases.

---

[17] http://www.amazon.com/Freedom-Eczema-Pool-Bethesda-1/dp/1491251336/ref=la_B00DRGNZLU_1_1_title_1_pap?s=books&ie=UTF8&qid=1387841174&sr=1-1
[18] Adapted from http://www.urmc.rochester.edu/Encyclopedia/Content.aspx?ContentTypeID=134&ContentID=123
[19] http://kidshealth.org/parent/general/body_basics/immune.html#

Stress has a tremendous impact on the immune system. Stress can corrupt our immune system. I will explain this in the next chapter.

Elevated Blood Sugars Weaken the Immune System

One last observation on the immune system. Did you know *Eating or drinking too much sugar curbs immune system cells that attack bacteria? This effect lasts for at least a few hours after downing a couple of sugary drinks.*[20]

Glucose exhausts immune cells. Glucose binds proteins on the surface of cells through a mechanism called glycosylation. Extra glucose in the blood of those with uncontrolled type 2 diabetes can result in glycosylated immune cells. These immune cells are activated in the absence of an infection and become exhausted and desensitized. Glycosylated immune cells are thus unable to respond effectively to infection and the immune system is weakened as a result.[21]

[20] http://www.webmd.com/cold-and-flu/10-immune-system-busters-boosters
[21] http://www.diabetesmonitor.com/education-center/diabetes-basics/elevated-blood-sugars-increase-risks-for-infections.htm

Chapter 3
A Word About Prescription Drugs and Medicine

Let me state from the start that I am not opposed to prescription drugs or the medical community. I thank God for the advances we have seen in both the medical and pharmaceutical fields. They have saved lives! Having said that however, prescription drugs may target relief, but they are not a cure, and in many cases can be a detrimental solution to your health issues. Have you ever listened to the commercials for different prescription drugs being marketed to the consumer today? They first tell you the wonderful benefits of their product and then a much longer list of potential side effects are recited. Many of the side effects listed are worse than the actual illness or disease being treated, to include death. We need to educate ourselves on the dangers of prescription drugs and be responsible for our health care. Let's look at some recent studies of healthcare and prescription drugs. This is not intended to frighten, but to educate.

According to The Institute of Medicine's study of the health care ("To Err is Human"[22]) system of 1999 and a follow up study by the New England Journal of Medicine in 2010[23], health care in the United States is not as safe as it could be.

---

[22] http://www.iom.edu/~/media/Files/Report%20Files/1999/To-Err-is-Human/To%20Err%20is%20Human%201999%20%20report%20brief.pdf
[23] http://www.nejm.org/doi/full/10.1056/NEJMsa1004404

Health care in the United States is not as safe as it should be--and can be. At least 44,000 people, and perhaps as many as 98,000 people, die in hospitals each year as a result of medical errors that could have been prevented, according to estimates from two major studies. Even using the lower estimate, preventable medical errors in hospitals exceed attributable deaths to such feared threats as motor-vehicle wrecks, breast cancer, and AIDS.[24]

These are just deaths in hospitals as a result of medical errors!

Types of Errors

Diagnostic
Error or delay in diagnosis
Failure to employ indicated tests
Use of outmoded tests or therapy
Failure to act on results of monitoring or testing

Treatment
Error in the performance of an operation, procedure, or test
Error in administering the treatment
Error in the dose or method of using a drug
Avoidable delay in treatment or in responding to an abnormal test
Inappropriate (not indicated) care

Preventive
Failure to provide prophylactic treatment
Inadequate monitoring or follow-up of treatment

---

[24] http://www.iom.edu/~/media/Files/Report%20Files/1999/To-Err-is-Human/To%20Err%20is%20Human%201999%20%20report%20brief.pdf

Other
Failure of communication
Equipment failure
Other system failure [25]

Just for comparison, all homicide deaths per year are about 16,259.[26] Accidental death by firearms in the U.S. per year are about 760. Fatal traffic crashes account for about 30,000 deaths per year.[27]

Now let's look at the number one cause of accidental death in the United States. Accidental prescription drug overdose.[28] According to the L.A. Times *"Prescription overdoses kill more people than heroin and cocaine. An L.A. Times review of coroners' records finds that drugs prescribed by a small number of doctors caused or contributed to a disproportionate number of deaths.*[29]

Perhaps you are thinking you don't have to worry as you won't overdose. How about the side effects of those same drugs?

Some Prescription Drugs for Acne and Their Side Effects (Not all side effects are listed)

This is not an exhaustive list of drugs used for Acne but a sampling. They all list possible side effects.

---

[25] SOURCE: Leape, Lucian; Lawthers, Ann G.; Brennan, Troyen A
[26] http://www.cdc.gov/nchs/fastats/homicide.htm
[27] http://www-fars.nhtsa.dot.gov/Main/index.aspx
[28] http://www.cnn.com/2012/11/14/health/gupta-accidental-overdose/
[29] http://www.latimes.com/news/science/prescription/la-me-prescription-deaths-20121111-html,0,2363903.htmlstory?main=true#ixzz2qy99qSGp

What are the possible side effects of Altinac, Atralin, Avita, Renova, Retin A Micro Gel, Retin-A, Tretin-X

Generic Name: tretinoin topical (Pronunciation: TRET in oin)

What are the possible side effects of tretinoin topical?[30]

Stop using this medication and get emergency medical help if you have any of these **signs of an allergic reaction:** *hives; difficulty breathing; swelling of your face, lips, tongue, or throat.*

Less serious side effects may include burning, warmth, stinging, tingling, itching, redness, swelling, dryness, peeling, irritation, or discolored skin.

This is not a complete list of side effects and others may occur.

What are the possible side effects of Korlym?[31]

Korlym

Korlym™

(mifepristone) 300 mg Tablets for Oral Use

WARNING

TERMINATION OF PREGNANCY

Mifepristone is a potent antagonist of progesterone and cortisol via the progesterone and glucocorticoid (GR-II) receptors, respectively. The antiprogestational effects will result in the termination of pregnancy. Pregnancy must therefore be excluded before the initiation of treatment with Korlym and

---

[30] http://www.rxlist.com/avita-drug/patient-images-side-effects.htm#sideeffects
[31] http://www.rxlist.com/korlym-side-effects-drug-center.htm

prevented during treatment and for one month after stopping treatment by the use of a non-hormonal medically acceptable method of contraception unless the patient has had a surgical sterilization, in which case no additional contraception is needed. Pregnancy must also be excluded if treatment is interrupted for more than 14 days in females of reproductive potential.[32]

The most frequently reported adverse reactions (reported in ≥ 20% of patients, regardless of relationship to Korlym) were nausea, fatigue, headache, decreased blood potassium, arthralgia, vomiting, peripheral edema, hypertension, dizziness, decreased appetite, and endometrial hypertrophy. Drug-related adverse events resulted in dose interruption or reduction in study drug in 40% of patients. The adverse reactions that occurred in ≥ 10% of the Cushing's syndrome patients receiving Korlym, regardless of relationship to Korlym, are shown in Table 1.[733]

Table 1: Treatment Emergent Adverse Events Occurring in ≥ 10% of Cushing's Syndrome Patients Receiving Korlym

BODY SYSTEM/ADVERSE REACTION	PERCENT (%) OF PATIENTS REPORTING EVENT (N = 50)
Gastrointestinal disorders	
Nausea	48
Vomiting	26
Dry mouth	18
Diarrhea	12

---

[32] http://www.rxlist.com/korlym-drug.htm
[33] http://www.rxlist.com/korlym-side-effects-drug-center.htm

Constipation	10

General disorders and administration/site conditions

Fatigue	48
Edema peripheral	26
Pain	14

Nervous system disorders

Headache	44
Dizziness	22
Somnolence	10

Musculoskeletal and connective tissue disorders

Arthralgia	30
Back pain	16
Myalgia	14
Pain in extremity	12

Investigations

Blood potassium decreased	34
Thyroid function test abnormal	18

Infections and infestations	
Sinusitis	14
Nasopharyngitis	12
Metabolism and nutrition disorders	
Decreased appetite	20
Anorexia	10
Vascular disorders	
Hypertension	24
Reproductive system and breast disorders	
Endometrial hypertrophy	38*
Respiratory, thoracic, and mediastinal disorders	
Dyspnea	16
Psychiatric disorders	
Anxiety	10

*The denominator was 26 females who had baseline and end-of-trial transvaginal ultrasound[34]

---

[34] http://www.rxlist.com/korlym-side-effects-drug-center.htm

What are the possible side effects of LOTRISONE®
(clotrimazole and betamethasone dipropionate) Cream LOTRISONE®
(clotrimazole and betamethasone dipropionate) Lotion

FOR TOPICAL USE ONLY. NOT FOR OPHTHALMIC, ORAL, OR INTRAVAGINAL USE. NOT RECOMMENDED FOR PATIENTS UNDER THE AGE OF 17 YEARS AND NOT RECOMMENDED FOR DIAPER DERMATITIS.?[35]

What are the possible side effects of betamethasone and clotrimazole topical ?[36]

*Get emergency medical help if you have any of these **signs of an allergic reaction:** hives; difficulty breathing; swelling of your face, lips, tongue, or throat. Stop using this medication and call your doctor at once if you have any of these signs that you may be absorbing betamethasone topical through your skin or gums:*

- *swelling, redness, or any signs of new infection;*
- *severe burning or stinging of treated skin;*
- *weight gain, rounding of the face;*
- *increased thirst or hunger, urinating more than usual; or*
- *anxiety, depressed mood.*
  Less serious side effects may include:

- *mild skin itching or irritation;*
- *dry skin;*
- *changes in skin color;*
- *increased acne; or*
- *scarring or thinning of the skin.*
  This is not a complete list of side effects and others may occur.

---

[35] http://www.rxlist.com/lotrisone-drug.htm
[36] http://www.rxlist.com/lotrisone-drug/patient-images-side-effects.htm

Drugs are Dangerous Whether Legal or Illegal

There are about 10,000 deaths per year from the effects of illegal drugs. But, according to an article in the *Journal of the American Medical Association (JAMA)* an estimated 106,000 hospitalized patients die each year from drugs which, by medical standards, are properly prescribed and properly administered. More than two million suffer serious side effects. [37]

Do You Know Someone Who Takes More Than One Prescription? Polypharmacy Is Increasingly Becoming a Health Concern For Many

"The average community-dwelling older adult takes 4.5 prescription drugs and 2.1 over-the-counter medications," *Dr. Stern reported. Polypharmacy is responsible for up to 28 percent of hospital admissions and, he added, if it were classified as such, it would be the fifth leading cause of death in the United States.*[38]

We need to keep in mind that there is always a risk of side effects every time we take a prescription drug. Not one of us, except those who intentionally overdose, expects that they will die by taking a medication. Unfortunately it not only can happen, but happens more often than most people realize. All prescription drugs have some negative side effects. The only way to avoid the risk from prescription drugs is to not take them. ***I am not suggesting you stop taking prescription drugs.*** Neither do I want you

---

[37] Lazarou J, Pomeranz BH, Corey PN: "Incidence of adverse drug reactions in hospitalized patients." JAMA 1998;279:1200.

[38]

http://www.nytimes.com/2007/09/18/health/18brod.html?ex=1347768000&en=1656caf314be267d&ei=5088&partner=rssnyt&emc=rss&_r=1&

to suffer from guilt if you do take medications that work for you. Self guilt can be one of the triggers for your particular disease or illness. I also know some who struggle with feeling they don't have faith if they take a prescription for a disease or illness. Here is my take on it. If the medication helps during your battle to overcome the disease or illness, utilize the relief until your victory is fully attained. My goal in providing the information in this chapter is to educate you to the fact that doctors and medicines are not the miracle workers. They have limitations. God on the other hand has no such limitations. He is the miracle worker. If we are violating spiritual laws, we will experience negative consequences. What I want to do is to provide healing alternatives that will deal with the violation of any spiritual roots that could be causing the disease or dis-ease in your life. Once those roots are dealt with, the fruit (dis-ease) will soon disappear.

Chapter 4
Stress, Fear and Anxiety

Doctors are not sure what exactly it is that causes a worsening of symptoms during mental stress. Atopic eczema patients commonly report that their symptoms are likely to get worse when they are mentally stressed. It is possible that a vicious cycle could develop - the symptoms of eczema stress the patient, the resulting stress exacerbates the symptoms, etc.[39] I believe the same can be said of those who suffer with acne as well.

In my research, I have found that stress, fear and anxiety play a major role in most all disease and illness, including acne. According to "Pathophysiology The Biologic Basis for Disease in Adults and Children 5th Edition" written and compiled by a number of professors, nurse practitioners, MDs, etc., *Psychologic stress may cause or exacerbate (worsen) several disease states, including many of the diseases (cardiovascular disease, cancer, and infectious diseases) implicated as the leading causes of death in the United States. Evidence also shows that stress is directly related to the cause of some diseases and conditions or at least affects the severity of symptoms and outcomes in a number of diseases and conditions, including irritable bowel syndrome, ulcers, asthma, autoimmune disorders, delayed wound healing,*

---

[39] http://www.medicalnewstoday.com/articles/14417.php

reproductive dysfunction, diabetes (worsening of symptoms), and depression.[40]

The most common sources of stress include family, social relationships, friends, work, and school.

Some examples of events causing stress would be problems at home, having a baby, losing a friend, preparing for tests or exams, vacation, losing or starting a job, deadlines, competition, being a perfectionist, lack of sleep, involvement in too many activities, being over your head in obligations, etc.

There is a correlation between acne and stress or fear which can relate but not be limited to conflict or relational issues. There can be other contributing factors, but emotional and relational conflict and stress are common contributors. These stressors can contribute to how a person feels about themselves. When you are experiencing negative thoughts about yourself, your serotonin levels begin to diminish. According to a recent study, lower serotonin levels are associated with early hardening of the arteries which can increase blood pressure.[41] Isn't it amazing how thoughts and emotions can impact our health?

Fear, Stress and Anxiety Can Be Real or Imagined

Some fears are not based in reality. There are fears concerning just about anything. Whether a fear is based in

---

[40] Pathophysiology: The Biologic Basis for Disease in Adults and Children 5th Edition ISBN:0323035078 page 311

[41] http://www.sciencedaily.com/releases/2006/03/060303205220.htm

reality or not, it is still a controlling presence in a person's life that needs to be conquered. Our society has learned to rename fear. We call it stress, anxiety, worry. Whenever I use the word fear, expand the definition to include stress and anxiety.

The Bible states that God has not given us a spirit of fear.[i] Fear is a spirit released against you to defeat you and hold you in captivity. How does it have access to your life? You come into agreement with it. Fear is an ungodly belief. Fear is not from God. Perfect love casts out all fear.[42] Fear is faith in the wrong direction. This is why in a later section of this book we will go through prayers to renounce involvement with fear, etc. They are the spiritual roots that lead to disease or illness.

Fear, Stress and Anxiety Creates Chemical Imbalance in the Brain

As stated earlier hypertension can actually be caused by ***emotional stress related to family and friends, work, or school. This is fear based.*** Fear, stress and anxiety can also cause an ***imbalance in brain chemicals, including serotonin.*** I would like to explore the fact that serotonin levels drop during stress and conflict with others or self. You begin to think wrongly about how you or others view you and the serotonin levels begin to drop. Medication or prescription drugs for depression or anxiety are given to boost serotonin levels. It is estimated that some 90% of our serotonin supply is

---

[42] 1 John 4:18 NKJV

found in the digestive tract and in blood platelets.[43] If this is true, is it any wonder that the serotonin levels begin to drop when we worry?

Serotonin is one of the main neurotransmitters in the brain. It is essential to the way the brain functions and processes information. According to Ohio clinical psychologist Joseph Carver, **stress greatly influences the levels of serotonin in the body. When a person experiences stress, serotonin is utilized at a higher than normal rate. Increased amounts of stress for prolonged periods of time can result in a depletion of serotonin**. *As levels continue to drop, it is harder for the body to replace them and maintain the necessary amounts needed to function efficiently.[44]*

Serotonin and the Immune System

There is also a link between serotonin and the immune system. According to the US National Library of Medicine, *5-HT (serotonin) is involved in interactions between the central nervous and immune systems.[45]*

By the way, some healing ministry research suggests that those who suffer with acne have the following in common; they battle with fear (as in stress and anxiety), have generational fear in their family history, worry about tomorrow, and have anger or hatred against self, others or God and a lack of trust of the same. As a result of the anger towards others or self (can be the result of peer pressure as

---

[43] http://www.webmd.com/depression/features/serotonin
[44] http://www.livestrong.com/article/127220-causes-low-serotonin/#ixzz2PQyVgyN7
[45] http://www.ncbi.nlm.nih.gov/pubmed/10080856

well), they may struggle with self-bitterness, self-hatred, rejection or self-rejection, guilt or condemnation. Those who suffer with cystic-acne (severe acne that manifests in cysts or nodules) tend to battle with fear of conflict that is primarily between two females or between close family members which can also lead to bitterness. Males can also be impacted. When you are not at peace with God, yourself and others, your body will respond. The fear can be a result of the conflict within yourself or with God or others and the stress that ensues. This conflict is internalized and produces the anger and/or guilt that can in turn cause hatred, self-hatred, rejection or self-rejection. Though we don't want to think of ourselves too highly, we also don't want to hate the person God has made. Have you ever said "I hate myself!" or "I hate when I do that!" or "I wish I had never been born!" or a host of other self-deprecating statements? If so, you battle self-hatred or self-rejection and it is damaging your health! These thoughts of hatred, self-hatred, rejection and self-rejection can then escalate within, causing a release of chemicals in the body or a reduction of those chemicals such as serotonin, the "feel good" body chemical. When serotonin is lacking, many are treated with anti-depressant medication. Anti-depressant medication can cause side effects such as high blood pressure (see my book Freedom From High Blood Pressure)[46]. To add to the problem, many medications for high blood pressure have the side effect of acid reflux.[47] (See my book "Freedom From Acid Reflux")[48] You can see

---

[46] http://www.amazon.com/Freedom-Blood-Pressure-Bethesda-Volume/dp/1489501444

[47] http://www.ncbi.nlm.nih.gov/pubmedhealth/PMH0001311/

[48] http://www.amazon.com/Freedom-From-Reflux-Robert-Campbell/dp/1491241314

the potential for too many prescriptions being given just to address the side effects of other prescription drugs while little energy is given to emotional causes and so the cycle continues. This certainly doesn't happen to everyone, but if you are in the cycle, this book can help. The key is to address the root issues so the cycle ceases.

We can see that a major factor in controlling acne is to maintain a healthy immune system. One of the key factors for a healthy immune system is to eliminate the stress, anxiety and fear in our life and/or relationships. When these emotions and mindsets are in play, they weaken the proper functioning of our immune system. These underlying issues in life are what I call spiritual roots.

As a side note, most doctors recommend therapy alongside the anti-depressant medications. The anti-depressants raise the serotonin levels so that a person can choose to have correct thoughts. Controlling negative emotions is the absolute solution as negative emotions throw the serotonin levels out of balance in the first place. The mind-body connection is real. We want to deal with root issues and not just medicate symptoms.

Chapter 5
Spiritual Roots to Disease

Before I explain more about the spiritual roots to disease, let me address the question of whether or not looking at spiritual roots to disease is Biblical. I believe there was an understanding in the Jewish culture that roots to disease did in fact exist. Though they may not have called them "spiritual roots", they did understand the connection of sin and sickness. For example in John 9:2, Jesus was asked, "who sinned, this man or his parents, that he was born this way?" It also states in Exodus 15:26 that if you obey the commandments, God will put none of the diseases of the Egyptians upon you. Jesus also told a man in John 5:14 to sin no more less a worse thing come upon you. We have lost this understanding in the church and so when we pray for the sick, we may see a miracle of healing and then a relapse, as the person healed did not change the behavior that contributed to the disease. If I have ulcers and do not deal with worry, I will not get lasting healing in my life. The best I can hope for is to medicate my disease which may not bring me 100% relief and I will have to deal with the side effects of that particular medication. This is why it is important to identify any spiritual roots to disease.

I have heard it said that the American Medical Association states that 80% of all incurable diseases have no biological cause. We have touched on some of the non biological causes to disease which would include stress, fear, anxiety, rejection and anger. We call these non biological causes to disease spiritual roots. When roots are dealt with the fruit of the roots is eliminated. Let's now look at how to get rid of the fruit of acne.

When I give you strategies to eliminate spiritual roots, I am getting this information based on research and case studies of individuals who suffer from acne, either from the medical community or healing centers. I gathered information from studies by the Mayo clinic and various other sources. I also found research and case studies of individuals from healing ministries who have worked with literally thousands of individuals over the years. As the case studies are examined, similar patterns of behavior, etc. are discovered with those who have the disease being studied.

I find it very encouraging to read of others involved in pursuing root issues related to the mind-body connection with disease or illness. One doctor has had incredible success in eliminating back pain for those who have herniated discs, the so called pinched nerve, and bone spurs all without surgery. Eighty eight percent of his patients have reported no more back pain, 10 percent reported improvement and only 2 percent reported no change. That is impressive! Here is the reason for his impressive statistics, he first interviews the patient to make sure they are receptive to TMS, Tension Myositis Syndrome, (characterized by psychogenic musculoskeletal and nerve symptoms) also known as mind-body syndrome. If they are open, he then begins with educating them to the mind-body connection. Though I don't agree with all of his conclusions, I believe he has discovered a Biblical root issue, negative spiritual and emotional activity.[49]

I also found this article from Northwestern Memorial Hospital that understands the importance in identifying the mind-body connection with ailments.

Chicago resident Anna Chapman had suffered from a mysterious pain for ten years. It started in her jaw and spread to her head, neck, and shoulders. Over time, the pain shot down her legs. She visited dozens of doctors and specialists, endured a number of tests and was misdiagnosed a handful of times. Just as Chapman thought she exhausted all other means of treatment, something clicked and she remembered hearing about TMS, Tension Myositis Syndrome, also known as mind-body syndrome. It was an epiphany that ultimately put Chapman back in control of her health and changed her life.

"The pain was awful. It forced me to give up on so many of the things I loved like gardening and playing tennis. Plus, on top of all the pain, the act of going to multiple doctors just to hear they don't know what's wrong with me was exhausting. It really took a toll on my life," said Chapman.

Chapman found John Stracks, MD, a family and integrative medicine physician with Northwestern Memorial Physicians Group who specializes in TMS. Stracks diagnosed Chapman with TMS affecting the

---

[49]http://www.tmswiki.org/ppd/An_Introduction_to_Tension_Myositis_Syndrome_(TMS)

muscles, ligaments, and nerves of the back and neck. The pain experienced with TMS is triggered by tension and, in most cases, can be eliminated by a mental process that involves focusing on the emotional, rather than the physical. Research increasingly supports the link between emotional and physical conditions, and scientists are now revealing how emotional signals can translate into physical pain. Back pain, neck pain, arthritis, migraine headaches, skin rashes, fibromyalgia, and many other conditions are caused or worsened by emotions such as tension, anger, fear, and grief.[50]

Let me give you an example of spiritual roots tied to a sickness or malady. Worry. Is this a medical problem or a spiritual problem? I contend it is a spiritual problem.

> *Psalms 37:8 Cease from anger, and forsake wrath; Do not fret — it only causes harm. NKJV*

Is this verse true? Yes. Does it speak to the problem? Yes. The problem is worry or fretting. What do we know about worry? It involves thoughts. These thoughts can lead to action or inaction, but they are just thoughts. What do these kind of thoughts produce in a person? These thoughts have the potential to cause ulcers. People who worry a lot tend to get ulcers. Is this an absolute? No, but it is common among ulcer sufferers. If they could eliminate the wrong thinking (spiritual roots), they could eliminate the ulcers.

Another example of a malady that can be caused by fear, stress, anxiety and anger is high blood pressure.

---

[50] http://www.nmh.org/nm/tms-diagnosis

Again, we would just be referring to thoughts, but they produce a negative impact in the body.

Let me continue briefly with the root of fear and how it impacts your body. As I stated earlier, fear in today's lifestyle includes worry, stress, anxiety, concerns, phobias, conflict with another person, perfectionism, etc. These are all fear based. Does this fear have any negative consequences in your body? Yes. Let me show you how.

Fear Is Sometimes Useful; Fight or Flight

Several bodily changes occur as a reaction to a fearful event. During fear, hormones that prepare us to adapt to stress are released in a chain reaction, first from the brain, which trigger in turn the release of stress hormones from the adrenal glands. Our heart rate increases, blood is redirected to body parts associated with fight or flight, and extra sugar is made available in the bloodstream via the liver.

Unresolved fear may convert to anxiety as we begin to grow accustomed to a threat. When we're anxious, the same physical changes that accompany fear occur at lower levels, with harmful effects on our body. Sustained increased heart output and constriction of blood vessels to rechannel blood to certain organs can contribute to the development of high blood pressure and cardiovascular disease. Altered sugar metabolism can worsen diabetes. The tendency for digestive activity to increase in times of stress can exacerbate underlying gastric ulcers.

Worry and anxiety involve recycling the same fear, repeatedly examining the outcomes and evaluating interventions. We sometimes use this activity to justify worry, assuming that repeated scrutiny will result in knowing what to do if worse comes to worst. This continual rehearsal of negative events in search of solutions may not benefit us should danger actually arise. The two thought processes, worry and planning, center in different parts of the brain. On magnetic resonance imaging, those who worry show activity in the emotional part of the brain, whereas those who plan show activity in the opposite hemisphere, the so-called logical half of the brain. This may mean that, from the standpoint of providing a good solution in the face of danger, worry is not the best strategy. Worry does not determine the best solution and move on to the next problem. It prevents us from detecting and dealing with new problems in a timely and effective way.

Physical symptoms of anxiety may include any of these: shortness of breath, sigh breathing, dry mouth, inability to swallow, trembling, weakness, incessant crying, circular or obsessive thoughts, inability to concentrate, paralytic or manic movements, insomnia, headache, recurrent nightmares, or extreme fatigue.

The Effect of Stress on the Immune System

The stress hormones released by the adrenals during episodes of fear and anxiety also affect white blood cells, the infection-fighting army within our blood. Initially, the surge of brain and adrenal hormones that accompanies stress causes an increase in circulating white blood cells. When cortisol remains high, however, white blood cell numbers are reduced. As stress, anxiety, or depression continue unabated over weeks or months, output of the adrenal hormone cortisol is consistently high and white blood cell numbers remain reduced.[51]

If we continually fear, our immune system degenerates and we get weaker and weaker and our health goes downhill. All this is based on thoughts that have impact in our body! Remember there is a connection between acne and the immune system. If you can eliminate what is compromising the immune system you can get freedom from acne.

I believe in most cases acne has a spiritual root (guilt, false-guilt, bitterness, self-bitterness, self-hatred, rejection, self-rejection, condemnation or fear) that manifests itself in the natural in our bodies, as explained previously.

Some believe that the chemicals released in our body determine what and how we think and feel. My contention is that our thoughts determine what is released in our bodies or what is depleted. Overcome the fear, worry, self-hatred, etc. and you can eliminate the negative chemical

---

[51] The preceding excerpt is taken from Chapter 12 of Colon & Rectal Cancer: A Comprehensive Guide for Patients & Families by Lorraine Johnston, copyright 2000 by O'Reilly & Associates, Inc.

releases and see your immune system function properly. This is what you can do to defeat acne. I believe the enemy of our soul learned long ago how to impact our bodies through wrong thinking such as fear, self-hatred, rejection, bitterness, etc.

Let's look at the roots of acne and overcome those roots so you can get closer to your cure. First I want to share an experience with you that involves my wife and migraines. She has not had acne, but many of the roots are the same or similar and I believe you can benefit from hearing how the knowledge of spiritual roots provided her cure.

Knowledge of Spiritual Roots Brings a Cure

My wife, Kathy, had been a sufferer of migraines (see my book Freedom From Migraines)[52], on occasion, for much of our married life. There were times she passed out because of the pain. We just accepted this as a part of her life with no real insight into what caused them. During her episodes she would need it to be dark and quiet and she would endure the migraine until it dissipated.

One night I came into the bedroom to get ready for a meeting we were both to attend and saw her suffering with another migraine. Because I had been researching healing methods from a Biblical perspective, I had come across an insight from Henry Wright in his book on fear. He made the following observation *"The psychogenic pain of*

---

[52] http://www.amazon.com/Freedom-Migraines-Pool-Bethesda-Healing-ebook/dp/B00CA36EYQ/ref=sr_1_1?s=books&ie=UTF8&qid=1387850000&sr=1-1&keywords=freedom+from+migraines+campbell

migraines produces real pain, which is caused by conflict with oneself out of a combination of fear and self-hatred... If you will get out of the spirit of Fear and get rid of the spirits of Self-Rejection, Self-Hatred, and Guilt, you will overcome migraine headaches.[ii]

I decided to put it to the test. This wasn't just a reciting of words, but a literal taking authority over the enemy who was plaguing my wife with migraines.

In my studies I had learned of my authority according to Luke 10:19 and how God had not given us a spirit of fear according to 2 Timothy 1:7, so I asked her if she had any guilt, self hatred, self rejection or fear. She couldn't think of anything and then I asked "What about false guilt?" After a couple minutes she said yes, she had false guilt. She had been condemning herself for not being able to help someone that she thought needed help. In reality there was nothing to feel guilty about as there was nothing that could have been done. This was obviously the enemy's trap set to snare her in an ungodly belief about herself and it had produced the desired effect. I led her in the process below (out loud) and the migraine dissipated. Since then we have used this process numerous times with the same results. I have also used it with others one on one and in group settings, such as during a seminar, and have gotten nearly 100 percent success! I believe the same results will hold true with acne.

Let's Look at the Spiritual Roots to Acne

Guilt is easy to understand and you are able to overcome it. With guilt, we just need to repent of wrong behavior and make it right between us, others and God. For example, if I have been lying, I need to ask God to forgive me, stop lying and make amends with those I have lied to or lied about. As a result, I have gotten rid of the guilt.

False guilt can be a little more tricky. False guilt can be the result of not meeting expectations. These can be either our own or someone else's expectations. Usually false guilt is the inner conflict of feeling disapproval from someone, even if that disapproval has not been expressed. I could be condemning myself mentally for not being able to do this or that, or wondering how someone feels about what I have or haven't done. This can be especially true if you grew up in a performance driven family where you had to perform in a certain way in order to get any approval.

Acne can also be caused by our being perfectionists (which is a form of fear of rejection and inner turmoil) and never being satisfied with ourselves or our efforts, which again creates false guilt. This can produce inner conflict, self rejection, condemnation and great inner turmoil.

The solution is to deal with any conflict with others or the inner conflict with self. If we can heal a relationship and make it right, we are to do so. *If it is possible, as far as it depends on you, live at peace with everyone.*[53]

---

[53] Romans 12:18 NIV

Chapter 6
The Law Of Agreement

There is power in agreement. In the garden of Eden, the enemies' strategy was to get Adam and Eve to come into agreement with him, for in so doing they would come out of agreement with God. When we come out of agreement with God, we lose all legal right to the benefits He provides us with. This is still the strategy of the enemy today. To come into agreement with the enemy and his kingdom values, is to come into agreement with ungodly beliefs. Whatsoever is not of faith is sin (Romans 14:23). Stress, fear and anxiety are ungodly beliefs. They did not exist in the garden of Eden before the fall. They are not part of the Kingdom of God.

Fear and faith both require us to believe something that has not yet happened. Fear and faith are both looking at the same circumstances but coming to different conclusions. One is faith based, the other fear based. Whatever you meditate on, you give power to become reality in your life. If we knew how powerful our thoughts were, we would think negatively less often. Fear is faith in the wrong direction. Many times we believe the doctors report over what God has said in His word. I look at the doctor's report as a prayer strategy to get victory over the disease I am battling.

> Job 3:25 For the thing I greatly feared has come upon me, And what I dreaded has happened to me. NKJV

Our authority is in our agreement with God. All the covenants are based on agreement. You walk in the blessings of the covenant by coming into agreement with it. You walk in the blessings of healing by coming into agreement with the promises of healing. The opposite is also true. If we come into agreement with stress, fear, anxiety, doubt and unbelief, we will be filled with sickness and disease (acne), insecurity, bitterness, etc. The enemy is a legalist. He has no power over us unless we have come into agreement with him in some area. I cannot exercise my authority over him if I am in agreement with him in any area of my life. Luke 10:19 says I have authority over all the power of the enemy, but, if I am holding onto unforgiveness, bitterness, etc., I will be unable to exercise that authority over him as I am in agreement with his kingdom values. Once I come out of agreement with the enemy, I have all authority over his power.

Remove the Legal Groundwork Beneath the Enemy's Feet

Our strategy for dealing with acne is to identify any agreement with the enemy and repent! Once we repent, we then come out of agreement, and exercise our authority over not only the enemy, but the disease afflicting us. One of the keys in exercising our authority is to speak to the mountain. In this case acne. There are many scriptures related to our words and what we say at the end of the book. This will make more sense as we go through the prayers and declarations concerning acne in the coming pages.

Let me remind you of what has been given to you as a follower of Jesus Christ. You have been given a gift of salvation. Many think of it as only the forgiveness of sins, but, it is so much more! Let's see what the Bible actually says.

Jesus Has Brought Us Salvation

> John 3:17 For God sent not his Son into the world to condemn the world; but that the world through him might be **saved** (Sozo). KJV

Strong's Number for saved is NT:4982 "Sozo" is used 109 times in the New Testament and means;

*To **save, deliver, make whole,** preserve safe from danger, loss, destruction, **deliverance from disease or demon possession, rescue of physical life from some impending peril or instant death, Of sick persons, to save from death and (by implication) to heal, restore to health; pass. to be healed, recover** (from The Complete Word Study Bible and The Complete Word Study Dictionary: New Testament Copyright © 1991, 1992, 1994, 2002 AMG International, Inc.)*

*To save, to keep safe and sound, to rescue from danger or destruction, to save a suffering one (from perishing), e. g. **one suffering from disease, to make well, heal, restore to health:** (from Thayer's Greek Lexicon, Electronic Database.*

> Hebrews 5:9 And being made perfect, he became the author of eternal **salvation** (Soteria) **unto all them that obey him**; KJV

Strong's Number for salvation is NT:4991 "Soteria" is used 46 times in the New Testament and means;

> *An acutely dynamic act in which gods or men snatch others by force from serious peril. "**to save from an illness," hence "to cure," not only "to be cured" but "to be or stay in good health**"; (from Theological Dictionary of the New Testament. Copyright © 1972-1989 By Wm. B. Eerdmans Publishing Co. All rights reserved.)*

> **deliverance, preservation, safety, salvation: deliverance from the molestation of enemies,** *(from Thayer's Greek Lexicon, PC Study Bible formatted Electronic Database. Copyright © 2006 by Biblesoft, Inc. All rights reserved.)*

This is what is yours as a follower of Jesus Christ! If we are ignorant of what is ours, we will not use or pursue those blessings and benefits. We will now look at the solutions that have benefited so many. As you exercise your authority, you are doing so from a place of authority as you are now in agreement with God!

If you are not yet a follower of Jesus Christ, do so today!

Matthew 11:28-30 Come to Me, all you who labor and are heavy laden, and I will give you rest. 29 Take My yoke upon you and learn from Me, for I am gentle and lowly in heart, and you will find rest for your souls. 30 For My yoke is easy and My burden is light." NKJV

Romans 3:23 for all have sinned and fall short of the glory of God, NKJV

Romans 3:10 As it is written: "There is none righteous, no, not one; NKJV

Romans 5:12 Therefore, just as through one man sin entered the world, and death through sin, and thus death spread to all men, because all sinned — NKJV

Romans 6:23 For the wages of sin is death, but the gift of God is eternal life in Christ Jesus our Lord. NKJV

Romans 5:8 But God demonstrates His own love toward us, in that while we were still sinners, Christ died for us. NKJV

Romans 10:9-10 that if you confess with your mouth the Lord Jesus and believe in your heart that God has raised Him from the dead, you will be saved. 10 For with the heart one believes unto righteousness, and with the mouth confession is made unto salvation. NKJV

Romans 10:13 For "whoever calls on the name of the Lord shall be saved."NKJV

2 Corinthians 5:17 Therefore, if anyone is in Christ, he is a new creation; old things have passed away; behold, all things have become new. NKJV

Romans 10:17 So then faith comes by hearing, and hearing by the word of God. NKJV

Chapter 7
Exercising Our Authority

The following is not a one-time event. Take these steps as often as necessary until your healing fully manifests. If the acne persists, do these steps again. You are re-training your mind and taking every thought captive by replacing ungodly beliefs with Godly beliefs. That is how you take every thought captive to the obedience of Christ!

How Do We Overcome Acne?

We Must Deal With Guilt, False Guilt, Self-bitterness, Self-Hatred, Self-Rejection, Condemnation, Fear (stress & anxiety), Self-Pity and The Spirit of Fear, Rejection and Condemnation.

1. **First of all you need to Recognize** whether or not you have any of the above. If you **have Guilt, False Guilt, Self-Bitterness, Self-Hatred, Self-Rejection, Self-Pity, Condemnation or Fear** (stress and anxiety) you can open yourself to **Spirits of Fear, Bitterness, Rejection, Self-Pity, and Condemnation** operating in your life. These can be passed down generationally in a family as a familiar spirit. We may see it as "that's just the way my family is." That may be true, but you don't have to continue believing that mindset any longer.

> *Psalms 51:6 Behold, You desire truth in the inward parts, And in the hidden part You will make me to know wisdom. NKJV*

2. Take **Responsibility** for your sin. After repenting of any known sin and asking for forgiveness and making restitution where necessary, genuine guilt is eliminated. Now you need to move on to the remaining roots. Agreeing with **False Guilt, Self-Bitterness, Self-Hatred, Self-Rejection, Self-Pity, Condemnation or Fear** is sin because it is an ungodly belief and a lack of trust of God. Don't blame others. Again, if you have legitimate guilt, repent and ask forgiveness for the sin causing the guilt. If you need to make something right with someone, do so.

Sometimes, before you can deal with a spiritual enemy, you need to remove the legal groundwork beneath his feet. This is where repentance comes in. An act that involves accurately judging yourself and owning where you are wrong.

Here's a trap: "all or nothing" thinking. Suppose you are mostly right and the other person is mostly wrong? What if you are 25% at fault but they are 75% at fault? Can you do a 25% repentance and reconciliation? No.

*But you can take 100% responsibility for your 25%....*and this often releases the GRACE on the *other person to own their 75%.*[54]

3. **Repent** and ask for forgiveness for any known sin. If you have agreed with **False Guilt, Self-Bitterness, Self-Hatred, Self-Rejection, Self-Pity, Condemnation, or Fear,** repent and ask God to forgive you. Ask God to forgive you for not trusting Him and for believing that your issues were beyond His reach, control, care or forgiveness. Ask for forgiveness from Him for believing He rejected you.

> *Psalms 32:3-6 When I refused to confess my sin, my body wasted away, and I groaned all day long. Day and night your hand of discipline was heavy on me. My strength evaporated like water in the summer heat. Finally, I confessed all my sins to you and stopped trying to hide my guilt. I said to myself, "I will confess my rebellion to the Lord ." And you forgave me! All my guilt is gone. Therefore, let all the godly pray to you while there is still time, that they may not drown in the floodwaters of judgment. NLT*

4. **Renounce (come out of agreement with)** involvement with **False Guilt, Self-bitterness, Self-Hatred, Self-Rejection, Self-Pity, Condemnation** or **Fear** and the **Spirits of Fear, Rejection, Self-Pity, Condemnation, and Bitterness** and command them to leave.

---

[54] http://lancelearning.biz/remove-the-legal-groundwork-beneath-your-enemys-feet/?inf_contact_key=80d982beeba6daacdcab647a8eb18ab07fb2dd5a9073cba4de7d315f5f0765e9

State you want nothing to do with **False Guilt**, **Self-bitterness**, **Self-Hatred**, **Self-Rejection**, **Self-Pity**, **Condemnation** or **Fear** and the **Spirits of Fear, Rejection, Self-Pity, Condemnation, and Bitterness** and command them to leave in Jesus' name.

5. **Resist** the sin of **False Guilt**, **Self-bitterness**, **Self-Hatred**, **Self-Rejection**, **Self-Pity**, **Condemnation** or **Fear** and all the enemy's strategies. He will attempt to get you to again agree with all the above. This is not a one-time battle over your thought life, but an on-going battle until you see victory! Flee from evil temptation, but pursue righteousness, faith, love and peace.[55]

6. **Reign** over your thought life. Don't allow these sins and ungodly beliefs to dominate your thought life any longer. Adopt a correct view of God. You need to see how willing and capable God is to keep all His promises to you. You also need to revise any false beliefs you have by examining what God says in His Word. Resist worldly values and beliefs contrary to the Word of God. We will provide Scriptures on specific topics at the end of this book. You are the one who takes every thought captive to the obedience of Christ. Believe God and trust His Word!

7. **Reestablish** your authority according to Luke 10:19 and 2 Timothy 1:7. You have authority over all the power of the enemy! Remember that **Spirits of Fear, Rejection, Self-Pity, Condemnation and Bitterness** come as a

---

[55] 2 Timothy 2:22 NKJV

result of agreement with their kingdom values of fear, rejection, condemnation and bitterness.

8. **Rest** in who God is. *God with us! A very present help in time of trouble.*[56] *Believe His promises! It is God who works in you both to will and to do of His good pleasure. Philippians 2:13*

9. Let the peace of God **Rule** and Reign in your heart by the Holy Spirit. Don't go back to worry and fear, false guilt, condemnation or rejection, but receive His peace on purpose!

10. **Speak** to **acne**. **Command** it to go and your body to be healed. Command all organs to function properly in Jesus' name. Command hormones to come into balance in Jesus' name. Command the serotonin levels to be restored to normal in Jesus' name. Command the arteries and blood vessels to function properly in Jesus' name. Command all pain to go in Jesus' name. Command all tissue to grow properly and to be restored in Jesus' name. Command all generational curses to be broken and command the **spirit of infirmity** to leave in Jesus' name. Command your immune system to be strengthened and to function properly in Jesus' name!

11. Be committed to **Rescuing** others by sharing these truths. This is not about trying to control others, but helping to empower them if they are open to it. The Scripture says ***Gently***!

---

56 Psalms 46:1 NKJV

> *2 Timothy 2:25-26 Gently instruct those who oppose the truth. Perhaps God will change those people's hearts, and they will learn the truth. 26 Then they will come to their senses and escape from the devil's trap. For they have been held captive by him to do whatever he wants. NLT*

> *Luke 10:19 Behold, I give you the authority to trample on serpents and scorpions, and over all the power of the enemy, and nothing shall by any means hurt you. NKJV*

I love the way it is worded in the Amplified Bible.

> *Luke 10:19 Behold! I have given you authority and power to trample upon serpents and scorpions, and [physical and mental strength and ability] over all the power that the enemy [possesses]; and nothing shall in any way harm you. AMP*

Luke 10:19 is your foundational Scripture. Memorize it!

Prayer
(It is important to remember this needs to be done out loud as the enemy does not know our thoughts. Our authority is expressed verbally. Jesus said "If you say to the mountain" Mark 11:23. These are not just words to be spoken, but they must also be mixed with faith and a confidence that God's word is true!)

Lord, forgive me for my sin. I repent of all known sin now. (List them to God) Forgive and cleanse me now.

Forgive me for agreeing with **False Guilt**, **Self-Bitterness**, **Self-Hatred**, **Self-Rejection**, **Self-Pity**, **Condemnation, Fear and Anxiety**. I acknowledge that **False Guilt**, **Self-bitterness**, **Self-Hatred**, **Self-Rejection**, **Self-Pity**, **Condemnation, Fear and Anxiety** is sin. I repent and turn away from **False Guilt**, **Self-Bitterness**, **Self-Hatred**, **Self-Rejection**, **Self-Pity**, **Condemnation, Fear and Anxiety** and the **Spirits of Fear, Rejection, Self-Pity, Condemnation, and Bitterness** now. I also ask that You forgive me for not trusting You Father. I know my lack of trusting You has grieved You. Forgive me. Wash me clean. Give me Your strength and ability to live free of **False Guilt**, **Self-bitterness**, **Self-Hatred**, **Self-Rejection**, **Self-Pity**, **Condemnation** and **Fear and Anxiety** in Jesus' name. I receive that strength and ability now. Where I have sinned against others, I will ask for their forgiveness and make restitution. I renounce all involvement with **False Guilt**, **Self-bitterness**, **Self-Hatred**, **Self-Rejection**, **Self-Pity**, **Condemnation, Fear and Anxiety** and the **Spirits of Fear, Rejection, Self-Pity, Condemnation, and Bitterness**. **False Guilt**, **Self-Bitterness**, **Self-Hatred**, **Self-Rejection**, **Self-Pity**, **Condemnation, Fear and Anxiety** and the **Spirits of Fear, Rejection, Self-Pity, Condemnation and Bitterness**, I want nothing to do with you any longer. I have authority over all of your power as I have been given that authority over you in Jesus' name according to Luke 10:19. I exercise that authority over you now. You have no legal right to be here as I have repented of agreement with you and so I command you to go now in Jesus' name. I break every generational curse in my life now in Jesus' name.

I now choose to resist all **False Guilt**, **Self-Bitterness**, **Self-Hatred**, **Self-Rejection**, **Self-Pity**, **Condemnation, Fear and Anxiety** and the **Spirits of Fear, Rejection, Self-Pity**, **Condemnation, and Bitterness** in Jesus' name from this time forth. I take authority over all thoughts to the obedience of Christ Jesus. **False Guilt**, **Self-bitterness**, **Self-Hatred**, **Self-Rejection**, **Self-Pity**, **Condemnation, Fear and Anxiety** will no longer dominate my thought life. God's Word will dominate my thought life from this time forth in Jesus' name. Thank You, Lord, that you are with me. Thank you for Your forgiveness and grace. Thank You for your peace. I receive Your **peace** even now. *(The definition of peace used by Jesus is health, welfare, prosperity and every kind of good.)* Jesus, I receive Your health, Your welfare, Your prosperity and every kind of good in Your name now!

I now take authority over acne. Acne go in Jesus' name. Spirit of infirmity go in Jesus' name! Serotonin levels come back to normal in Jesus' name. Arteries function properly in Jesus' name. Immune system be strengthened and made whole and function properly in Jesus' name! Female organs function properly in Jesus' name. Tissue grow properly in Jesus' name and be restored. Hormones come into balance in Jesus' name! I command all pain and acne to go now in Jesus' name! Thank You, Lord, that You have forgiven me all my iniquities and You have healed all my diseases. Thank You for my healing now in Jesus' name.

> *Psalms 103:1-5 Bless the Lord, O my soul; And all that is within me, bless His holy name! 2 Bless the Lord, O my soul, And forget not all His benefits: 3 Who forgives all your iniquities, Who heals all your diseases, 4 Who redeems your life from destruction, Who crowns you with lovingkindness and tender mercies, 5 Who satisfies your mouth with good things, So that your youth is renewed like the eagle's. NKJV*

My Prayer For You

Father, I thank you for releasing Your healing grace to this child that You love right now in Jesus' name. According to Luke 10:19, I take authority over all afflicting and hindering spirits in the name of Jesus and command them to loose their hold and go now in Jesus' name. I command the spirits of Fear, Rejection, Self-Pity, Bitterness and Condemnation to loose their hold and go now in Jesus' name! I command the spirit of infirmity to loose its hold now and to go in Jesus' name. I take authority over every generational spirit and curse and command them to go in Jesus' name. I command all pain to go now in Jesus' name! Self-Rejection go! Self-Hatred go! Self-Pity go! Condemnation go! False-Guilt go! Fear go! I command all organs to function properly and all hormones to come into balance now in Jesus' name. I command acne to loose it's hold and go now! I speak a word of restoration over all damage in this body and for healing virtue to flow now in Jesus' name. I speak to the immune system and command it to be healed and restored now in Jesus' name. Healing virtue and peace come now in Jesus' name I pray, amen.

Your Daily Declaration (Spoken out loud based on *Job 22:28 "You will also decree a thing, and it will be established for you; And light will shine on your ways. NASB)*

I am accepted in the beloved. I am loved and cared for by God and I am His workmanship. I have authority over all the power of the enemy and nothing shall by any means hurt me. No weapon formed against me shall prosper in Jesus' name. All fear has gone and I have power, love and a sound mind. I am prospering and enjoying good health even as my soul prospers. My serotonin levels are normal and my immune system is functioning properly in Jesus' name. By Jesus stripes I am healed. I receive His strength and restoration into my life and body now. My body is being made new!

Chapter 8
Maintaining Freedom

The following are adapted from the "Steps To Freedom In Christ" by Neil Anderson.

To maintain freedom commit to the following;

1. **Seek legitimate Christian fellowship** where you can walk in the light and speak the truth in love, where you will be supported in walking out your healing and wholeness.

2. **Renew** your mind by washing it with the Word of God. Study your Bible daily. Memorize key verses. This is how our minds are renewed.

> *Ephesians 5:26 that He might sanctify and cleanse her (the Church) with the washing of water by the word, NKJV*

3. **Realize** who you are in Christ. Christ in you does not fear or worry!

> *Galatians 2:20 I have been crucified with Christ [in Him I have shared His crucifixion]; it is no longer I who live, but Christ (the Messiah) lives in me; and the life I now live in the body I live by faith in (by adherence to and reliance on and complete trust in) the Son of God, Who loved me and gave Himself up for me. AMP*

4. **Reign** over your thought life. Take every thought captive to the obedience of Christ. Assume responsibility for your thought life, reject the lie, choose the truth and stand firm in your position in Christ. Do this daily! Review teachings in this book to remind yourself of the truth in order to walk out your healing and wholeness. Don't drift away! It is very easy to get lazy in your thoughts and revert back to old habit patterns of thinking. Share your struggles openly with a trusted friend. You need at least one friend who will stand with you. Take Every Thought Captive!

> *2 Corinthians 10:5 [Inasmuch as we] refute arguments and theories and reasonings and every proud and lofty thing that sets itself up against the [true] knowledge of God; and we lead every thought and purpose away captive into the obedience of Christ (the Messiah, the Anointed One), AMP*

5. **Rest** in who God is. God with you!

> *1 John 4:18 There is no fear in love; but perfect love casts out fear, because fear involves torment. But he who fears has not been made perfect in love. NKJV*

> *Matthew 1:23 "Behold, the virgin shall be with child, and bear a Son, and they shall call His name Immanuel,"* which is translated, "God with us." NKJV*

> *Philippians 4:13 I can do all things through Christ* who strengthens me. NKJV*

6. **Resist** fear and worry. In order for the devil to flee, we need to resist. Nothing comes without warfare. He will try and come back, but you must resist him.

James 4:7-8 Therefore submit to God. Resist the devil and he will flee from you. 8 Draw near to God and He will draw near to you. Cleanse your hands, you sinners; and purify your hearts, you double-minded. NKJV

7. Let the peace of God **Rule** and Reign in your heart by the Holy Spirit. Invite that peace to come now. The word peace means health, welfare, prosperity and every kind of good!

*Colossians 3:15 And let the peace (soul harmony which comes) from Christ rule (act as umpire continually) in your hearts [deciding and settling with finality all questions that arise in your minds, in that peaceful state] to which as [members of Christ's] one body you were also called [to live]. And be thankful (appreciative), [giving praise to God always]. AMP **Peace=Health, welfare, prosperity and every kind of good!***

*Romans 15:13 Now may the God of hope fill you with all joy and peace in believing, that you may abound in hope by the power of the Holy Spirit. NKJV **Peace=Health, welfare, prosperity and every kind of good!***

8. **Renounce** involvement with **False Guilt**, **Self-bitterness**, **Self-Hatred**, **Self-Rejection**, **Condemnation, Fear and Anxiety** and the **Spirits of Fear, Rejection, Condemnation and Bitterness** if you stumble. In the book of Acts there were those who were involved in magic (a forbidden practice) and as a sign of repentance they brought all their books on magic and they burned (renounced) those books publicly, so we renounce all involvement with **False Guilt**, **Self-bitterness**, **Self-Hatred**, **Self-Rejection**, **Condemnation, Fear and Anxiety** and the **Spirits of Fear, Rejection, Condemnation and Bitterness**.

9. **Don't expect another person to fight your battle for you.** Others can help, but they can't think, pray, read the Bible or choose the truth for you.

Chapter 9
Key Scriptures for Victory

Meditate on and apply these verses to your life. If you need to repent in an area, do so and take up your God given authority over all **Fear (stress & anxiety), Anger (possible fits of rage), Rejection, Bitterness, Self-Bitterness, Self-Hatred, Self-Rejection and Condemnation** Self-Hatred, Self-Rejection, Condemnation, Fear, Worry and Stress!

> *2 Timothy 3:16 All Scripture is given by inspiration of God, and is profitable for doctrine, for reproof, for correction, for instruction in righteousness, NKJV*

God's Faithfulness

God cares for me ~

> *Deuteronomy 7:9 "Therefore know that the Lord your God, He is God, the faithful God who keeps covenant and mercy for a thousand generations with those who love Him and keep His commandments; NKJV*

God is faithful and compassionate ~

> *Lamentations 3:22-23 Through the Lord 's mercies we are not consumed, Because His compassions fail not. 23 They are new every morning; Great is Your faithfulness. NKJV*

God comforts me in my darkest times ~

> *Job 35:10 But no one says, 'Where is God my Maker, Who gives songs in the night, NKJV*

God watches over me ~

> *Psalms 12:5 "For the oppression of the poor, for the sighing of the needy, Now I will arise," says the Lord; "I will set him in the safety for which he yearns." NKJV*

God comforts me ~

> *Isaiah 40:9-11 O Zion, You who bring good tidings, Get up into the high mountain; O Jerusalem, You who bring good tidings, Lift up your voice with strength, Lift it up, be not afraid; Say to the cities of Judah, "Behold your God!" 10 Behold, the Lord God shall come with a strong hand, And His arm shall rule for Him; Behold, His reward is with Him, And His work before Him. 11 He will feed His flock like a shepherd; He will gather the lambs with His arm, And carry them in His bosom, And gently lead those who are with young. NKJV*

God promises to comfort me when I mourn ~

> *Matthew 5:4 Blessed are those who mourn, For they shall be comforted. NKJV*

God's Holy Spirit is my Comforter ~

> *John 14:16 And I will pray the Father, and He will give you another Helper, that He may abide with you forever — NKJV*

God gives power to me ~

> *Isaiah 40:29 He gives power to the weak, And to* those who have *no might He increases strength. NKJV*

God is my refuge and fortress ~

> *Psalms 91 He who dwells in the secret place of the Most High Shall abide under the shadow of the Almighty. 2 I will say of the Lord , "He is my refuge and my fortress; My God, in Him I will trust." 3 Surely He shall deliver you from the snare of the fowler And from the perilous pestilence. 4 He shall cover you with His feathers, And under His wings you shall take refuge; His truth* shall be your *shield and buckler. 5 You shall not be afraid of the terror by night,* Nor *of the arrow* that *flies by day, 6* Nor *of the pestilence* that *walks in darkness,* Nor *of the destruction* that *lays waste at noonday. 7 A thousand may fall at your side, And ten thousand at your right hand;* But *it shall not come near you. 8 Only with your eyes shall you look, And see the reward of the wicked. 9 Because you have made the Lord , who is my refuge, Even the Most High, your dwelling place, 10 No evil shall befall you, Nor shall any plague come near your dwelling; 11 For He*

> shall give His angels charge over you, To keep you in all your ways. 12 In their hands they shall bear you up, Lest you dash your foot against a stone. 13 You shall tread upon the lion and the cobra, The young lion and the serpent you shall trample underfoot. 14 "Because he has set his love upon Me, therefore I will deliver him; I will set him on high, because he has known My name. 15 He shall call upon Me, and I will answer him; I will be with him in trouble; I will deliver him and honor him. 16 With long life I will satisfy him, And show him My salvation." NKJV

God is my sufficiency ~

> II Corinthians 3:5 Not that we are sufficient of ourselves to think of anything as being from ourselves, but our sufficiency is from God, KJV

I am more than a conqueror ~

> Romans 8:37 Yet in all these things we are more than conquerors through Him who loved us. NKJV

God gives us the will and ability to do His will ~

> Philippians 2:13 for it is God who works in you both to will and to do for His good pleasure. NKJV

God's Acceptance of You

He has made me a highly favored one ~

Ephesians 1:3-6 Blessed be the God and Father of our Lord Jesus Christ, who has blessed us with every spiritual blessing in the heavenly places in Christ, 4 just as He chose us in Him before the foundation of the world, that we should be holy and without blame before Him in love, 5 having predestined us to adoption as sons by Jesus Christ to Himself, according to the good pleasure of His will, 6 to the praise of the glory of His grace, by which He made us accepted (highly favored one) in the Beloved. NKJV

I am God's child by His adoption ~

Romans 8:15-17 For you did not receive the spirit of bondage again to fear, but you received the Spirit of adoption by whom we cry out, "Abba, Father." 16 The Spirit Himself bears witness with our spirit that we are children of God, 17 and if children, then heirs — heirs of God and joint heirs with Christ, if indeed we suffer with Him, that we may also be glorified together. NKJV

Christ has received me and adopted me as His child~

Romans 15:7 Therefore receive one another, just as Christ also received us, to the glory of God. NKJV

> *Psalms 27:10 Although my father and my mother have forsaken me, yet the Lord will take me up [adopt me as His child]. AMP*

> *Psalms 94:14 For the Lord will not cast off His people, Nor will He forsake His inheritance. NKJV*

He will never leave or forsake me ~

> *Hebrews 13:5 Let your conduct be without covetousness; be content with such things as you have. For He Himself has said, "I will never leave you nor forsake you." NKJV*

> *Deuteronomy 31:6 Be strong and of good courage, do not fear nor be afraid of them; for the Lord your God, He is the One who goes with you. He will not leave you nor forsake you." NKJV*

My Victory

No weapon formed against me shall prosper ~

> *Isaiah 54:17 No weapon formed against you shall prosper, And every tongue which rises against you in judgment You shall condemn. This is the heritage of the servants of the Lord, And their righteousness is from Me," Says the Lord. NKJV*

I will live a long life ~

> *Psalms 91:16 With long life will I satisfy him and show him My salvation. NKJV*

I have the right self-talk ~

> *Psalms 103:1-5 Bless the Lord, O my soul; And all that is within me, bless His holy name! Bless the Lord, O my soul, And forget not all His benefits: Who forgives all your iniquities, Who heals all your diseases, Who redeems your life from destruction, Who crowns you with lovingkindness and tender mercies, Who satisfies your mouth with good things, So that your youth is renewed like the eagle's. NKJV*

What I Say Matters

> *Proverbs 18:21 Death and life are in the power of the tongue, and they who indulge in it shall eat the fruit of it [for death or life]. AMP*

> *Proverbs 18:4 The words of a [discreet and wise] man's mouth are like deep waters [plenteous and difficult to fathom], and the fountain of skillful and godly Wisdom is like a gushing stream [sparkling, fresh, pure, and life- giving]. AMP*

Proverbs 10:20-21 The tongues of those who are upright and in right standing with God are as choice silver; the minds of those who are wicked and out of harmony with God are of little value. The lips of the [uncompromisingly] righteous feed and guide many, but fools die for want of understanding and heart. AMP

Proverbs 10:31 The mouths of the righteous (those harmonious with God) bring forth skillful and godly Wisdom, but the perverse tongue shall be cut down [like a barren and rotten tree]. AMP

Matthew 12:35-37 The good man from his inner good treasure flings forth good things, and the evil man out of his inner evil storehouse flings forth evil things. But I tell you, on the day of judgment men will have to give account for every idle (inoperative, nonworking) word they speak. For by your words you will be justified and acquitted, and by your words you will be condemned and sentenced. AMP

Ephesians 4:29 Let no foul or polluting language, nor evil word nor unwholesome or worthless talk [ever] come out of your mouth, but only such [speech] as is good and beneficial to the spiritual progress of others, as is fitting to the need and the occasion, that it may be a blessing and give grace (God's favor) to those who hear it. AMP

Proverbs 4:23 Guard your heart above all else, for it determines the course of your life. NLT

Colossians 4:6 Let your speech at all times be gracious (pleasant and winsome), seasoned [as it were] with salt, [so that you may never be at a loss] to know how you ought to answer anyone [who puts a question to you]. AMP

My Victory Is Connected To My Obedience To God's Word

Leviticus 26:14-22 "But if you will not listen to me and will not do all these commandments, if you spurn my statutes, and if your soul abhors my rules, so that you will not do all my commandments, but break my covenant, then I will do this to you: I will visit you with panic, with wasting disease and fever that consume the eyes and make the heart ache. And you shall sow your seed in vain, for your enemies shall eat it. I will set my face against you, and you shall be struck down before your enemies. Those who hate you shall rule over you, and you shall flee when none pursues you. And if in spite of this you will not listen to me, then I will discipline you again sevenfold for your sins, and I will break the pride of your power, and I will make your heavens like iron

> *and your earth like bronze. And your strength shall be spent in vain, for your land shall not yield its increase, and the trees of the land shall not yield their fruit. "Then if you walk contrary to me and will not listen to me, I will continue striking you, sevenfold for your sins. And I will let loose the wild beasts against you, which shall bereave you of your children and destroy your livestock and make you few in number, so that your roads shall be deserted. ESV*

Anger

I will not let the sun go down on my wrath~

> *Ephesians 4:26-27 "Be angry, and do not sin": do not let the sun go down on your wrath, 27 nor give place to the devil. NKJV*

I will be slow to get angry~

> *James 1:19-20 So then, my beloved brethren, let every man be swift to hear, slow to speak, slow to wrath; 20 for the wrath of man does not produce the righteousness of God. NKJV*

I will be slow to speak~

> *Proverbs 29:11 A fool vents all his feelings, But a wise man holds them back. NKJV*

My anger does not produce righteousness~

> *James 1:20 for the wrath of man does not produce the righteousness of God. NKJV*

I am slow to anger~

> *Proverbs 19:11 The discretion of a man makes him slow to anger, And his glory is to overlook a transgression. NKJV*

I will cease from anger~

> *Psalms 37:8 Cease from anger, and forsake wrath; Do not fret — it only causes harm. NKJV*

Outbursts of wrath are works of the flesh~

> *Galatians 5:19-20 Now the works of the flesh are evident, which are: adultery, fornication, uncleanness, lewdness, 20 idolatry, sorcery, hatred, contentions, jealousies, outbursts of wrath, selfish ambitions, dissensions, heresies, NKJV*

I will treat others as I want to be treated~

> *Luke 6:31 And just as you want men to do to you, you also do to them likewise. NKJV*

I am slow to anger and rule my spirit~

> *Proverbs 16:32 He who is slow to anger is better than the mighty, And he who rules his spirit than he who takes a city. NKJV*

I put off anger and wrath~

> *Colossians 3:8 But now you yourselves are to put off all these: anger, wrath, malice, blasphemy, filthy language out of your mouth. NKJV*

Anger rests in fools~

> *Ecclesiastes 7:9 Do not hasten in your spirit to be angry, For anger rests in the bosom of fools. NKJV*

Fear

God is my shield to protect me ~

> *Genesis 15:1 After these things the word of the Lord came to Abram in a vision, saying, "Do not be afraid, Abram. I am your shield, your exceedingly great reward." NKJV*

Because I fear the Lord He teaches me ~

> *Psalms 25:12 Who is the man that fears the Lord? Him shall He teach in the way He chooses. NKJV*

God watches over me, I will not fear ~

> *Psalms 91:5 You shall not be afraid of the terror by night, Nor of the arrow that flies by day, NKJV*

I do not need to fear bad news ~

> *Psalms 112:7 He will not be afraid of evil tidings; His heart is steadfast, trusting in the Lord. NKJV*

God is with me and strengthens and upholds me ~

Isaiah 41:10 Fear not, for I am with you; Be not dismayed, for I am your God. I will strengthen you, Yes, I will help you, I will uphold you with My righteous right hand.' NKJV

God will help me ~

Isaiah 41:13 For I, the Lord your God, will hold your right hand, Saying to you, 'Fear not, I will help you.' NKJV

My sleep will be sweet for God is my confidence ~

Proverb 3:24-26 When you lie down, you will not be afraid; Yes, you will lie down and your sleep will be sweet. 25 Do not be afraid of sudden terror, Nor of trouble from the wicked when it comes; 26 For the Lord will be your confidence, And will keep your foot from being caught. NKJV

I have power, love and a sound mind ~

II Tim 1:7 For God has not given us a spirit of fear, but of power and of love and of a sound mind. NKJV

God is my Father ~

Romans 8:15 For you did not receive the spirit of bondage again to fear, but you received the Spirit of adoption by whom we cry out, "Abba, Father." NKJV

God will never leave or forsake me ~

> *Hebrews 13:5-6 Let your conduct be without covetousness; be content with such things as you have. For He Himself has said, "I will never leave you nor forsake you." 6 So we may boldly say: "The Lord is my helper; I will not fear. What can man do to me?" NKJV*

The Lord is the strength of my life ~

> *Psalms 27:1 The Lord is my light and my salvation; Whom shall I fear? The Lord is the strength of my life; Of whom shall I be afraid? NKJV*

God delivers me of all my fears ~

> *Psalms 34:4 I sought the Lord , and He heard me, And delivered me from all my fears. NKJV*

God is very present and helps me in times of trouble~

> *Psalms 46:1-3 God is our refuge and strength, A very present help in trouble. 2 Therefore we will not fear, Even though the earth be removed, And though the mountains be carried into the midst of the sea; 3 Though its waters roar and be troubled, Though the mountains shake with its swelling. NKJV*

Whenever I go through difficulty God is with me ~

> *Isaiah 43:1-2 But now, thus says the Lord , who created you, O Jacob, And He who formed you, O Israel: "Fear not, for I have redeemed you; I have called you by your name; You are Mine. 2 When you pass through the waters, I will be with you; And through the rivers, they shall not overflow you. When you walk through the fire, you shall not be burned, Nor shall the flame scorch you. NKJV*

I listen to the Lord and dwell safely ~

> *Proverb 1:33 But whoever listens to me will dwell safely, And will be secure, without fear of evil." NKJV*

God is my helper ~

> *Hebrews 13:6 So we may boldly say: "The Lord is my helper; I will not fear. What can man do to me?" NKJV*

God's love drives away fear ~

> *1 John 4:18 There is no fear in love; but perfect love casts out fear, because fear involves torment. But he who fears has not been made perfect in love. NKJV*

Worry and Anxiety

I will not worry, God will take care of me ~

Matthew 6:25-34 "Therefore I say to you, do not worry about your life, what you will eat or what you will drink; nor about your body, what you will put on. Is not life more than food and the body more than clothing? 26 Look at the birds of the air, for they neither sow nor reap nor gather into barns; yet your heavenly Father feeds them. Are you not of more value than they? 27 Which of you by worrying can add one cubit to his stature? 28 "So why do you worry about clothing? Consider the lilies of the field, how they grow: they neither toil nor spin; 29 and yet I say to you that even Solomon in all his glory was not arrayed like one of these. 30 Now if God so clothes the grass of the field, which today is, and tomorrow is thrown into the oven, will He not much more clothe you, O you of little faith? 31 "Therefore do not worry, saying, 'What shall we eat?' or 'What shall we drink?' or 'What shall we wear?' 32 For after all these things the Gentiles seek. For your heavenly Father knows that you need all these things. 33 But seek first the kingdom of God and His righteousness, and all these things shall be added to you. 34 Therefore do not worry about tomorrow, for tomorrow will worry about its own things. Sufficient for the day is its own trouble. NKJV

I trust in my God and I have peace ~

> *Isaiah 26:3 You will keep him in perfect peace, Whose mind is stayed on You, Because he trusts in You. NKJV*

I cast my burden on the Lord and He sustains me ~

> *Psalms 55:22 Cast your burden on the Lord , And He shall sustain you; He shall never permit the righteous to be moved. NKJV*

I will make my requests known to God in prayer with a thankful heart ~

> *Philippians 4:6-7 Be anxious for nothing, but in everything by prayer and supplication, with thanksgiving, let your requests be made known to God; 7 and the peace of God, which surpasses all understanding, will guard your hearts and minds through Christ Jesus. NKJV*

Because I love God all things work out to my good ~

> *Romans 8:28 And we know that all things work together for good to those who love God, to those who are the called according to His purpose. NKJV*

I have the peace of Jesus which is translated (health, welfare, prosperity and every kind of good) ~

> *John 14:27 Peace I leave with you, My peace I give to you; not as the world gives do I give to you. Let not your heart be troubled, neither let it be afraid. NKJV*

I will not worry about what I should say as He will teach me what to say ~

> *Luke 12:11-12 "Now when they bring you to the synagogues and magistrates and authorities, do not worry about how or what you should answer, or what you should say. 12 For the Holy Spirit will teach you in that very hour what you ought to say." NKJV*

I cast my cares on Him ~

> *I Peter 5:7 casting all your care upon Him, for He cares for you. NKJV*

I am full of courage because He has strengthened my heart ~

> *Psalms 31:24 Be of good courage, And He shall strengthen your heart, All you who hope in the Lord. NKJV*

> *Psalms 27:14 Wait on the Lord; Be of good courage, And He shall strengthen your heart; Wait, I say, on the Lord ! NKJV*

Forgiveness

God forgives my many sins ~

> *Psalms 65:3 When we were overwhelmed by sins,*
> *you forgave our transgressions. NIV*

God forgives me because He loves me ~

> *Psalms 86:50 For You, Lord, are good, and ready to*
> *forgive, And abundant in mercy to all those who call*
> *upon You. NKJV*

God makes me as clean as freshly fallen snow ~

> *Isaiah 1:18 "Come now, and let us reason together,"*
> *Says the Lord, "Though your sins are like scarlet,*
> *They shall be as white as snow; Though they are red*
> *like crimson, They shall be as wool. NKJV*

God removes my impurities ~

> *Ezekiel 36:25 Then I will sprinkle clean water on*
> *you, and you shall be clean; I will cleanse you from*
> *all your filthiness and from all your idols. NKJV*

I must forgive others ~

> *Matthew 6:14-15 14 "For if you forgive men their*
> *trespasses, your heavenly Father will also forgive*
> *you. 15 But if you do not forgive men their*
> *trespasses, neither will your Father forgive your*
> *trespasses. NKJV*

I cannot keep track of how many times I have
forgiven ~

> *Matthew 18:21-35 Then Peter came to Him and said,*
> *"Lord, how often shall my brother sin against me,*
> *and I forgive him? Up to seven times?" 22 Jesus said*
> *to him, "I do not say to you, up to seven times, but*
> *up to seventy times seven. 23 Therefore the*
> *kingdom of heaven is like a certain king who wanted*
> *to settle accounts with his servants. 24 And when he*
> *had begun to settle accounts, one was brought to*
> *him who owed him ten thousand talents. 25 But as*
> *he was not able to pay, his master commanded that*
> *he be sold, with his wife and children and all that he*
> *had, and that payment be made. 26 The servant*
> *therefore fell down before him, saying, 'Master,*
> *have patience with me, and I will pay you all.' 27*
> *Then the master of that servant was moved with*
> *compassion, released him, and forgave him the debt.*
> *28 "But that servant went out and found one of his*
> *fellow servants who owed him a hundred denarii;*
> *and he laid hands on him and took him by the*
> *throat, saying, 'Pay me what you owe!' 29 So his*
> *fellow servant fell down at his feet and begged him,*
> *saying, 'Have patience with me, and I will pay you*
> *all.' 30 And he would not, but went and threw him*
> *into prison till he should pay the debt. 31 So when*
> *his fellow servants saw what had been done, they*
> *were very grieved, and came and told their master*
> *all that had been done. 32 Then his master, after he*
> *had called him, said to him, 'You wicked servant! I*
> *forgave you all that debt because you begged me.*

33 Should you not also have had compassion on your fellow servant, just as I had pity on you?' 34 And his master was angry, and delivered him to the torturers until he should pay all that was due to him. 35 "So My heavenly Father also will do to you if each of you, from his heart, does not forgive his brother his trespasses." NKJV

I must freely forgive others as God has forgiven me ~

Colossians 3:13 bearing with one another, and forgiving one another, if anyone has a complaint against another; even as Christ forgave you, so you also must do. NKJV

God will forgive my sins as I confess them ~

1 John 1:8-9 If we say that we have no sin, we deceive ourselves, and the truth is not in us. 9 If we confess our sins, He is faithful and just to forgive us our sins and to cleanse us from all unrighteousness. NKJV

God has removed my sins from me ~

Psalms 103:12 As far as the east is from the west, So far has He removed our transgressions from us. NKJV

God will remember my sins no more ~

Hebrews 8:12 For I will be merciful to their unrighteousness, and their sins and their lawless deeds I will remember no more." NKJV

God casts my sins into the depths of the sea ~

> *Micah 7:19 He will again have compassion on us, And will subdue our iniquities. You will cast all our sins Into the depths of the sea. NKJV*

God has cast my sins behind His back~

> *Isaiah 38:17 Indeed it was for my own peace That I had great bitterness; But You have lovingly delivered my soul from the pit of corruption, For You have cast all my sins behind Your back. NKJV*

God does not remember my sins~

> *Isaiah 43:25 "I, even I, am He who blots out your transgressions for My own sake; And I will not remember your sins. NKJV*

Because I am in Christ, all things are new~

> *2 Corinthians 5:17 Therefore, if anyone is in Christ, he is a new creation; old things have passed away; behold, all things have become new. NKJV*

Thoughts

My thoughts must be guarded as sin starts with a thought ~

> *Matthew 5:27-30 "You have heard that it was said to those of old, 'You shall not commit adultery.' 28 But I say to you that whoever looks at a woman to lust for her has already committed adultery with her in his heart. 29 If your right eye causes you to sin, pluck it out and cast it from you; for it is more profitable for you that one of your members perish, than for your whole body to be cast into hell. 30 And if your right hand causes you to sin, cut it off and cast it from you; for it is more profitable for you that one of your members perish, than for your whole body to be cast into hell. NKJV*

My mind is being transformed and renewed ~

> *Romans 12:2 And do not be conformed to this world, but be transformed by the renewing of your mind, that you may prove what is that good and acceptable and perfect will of God. NKJV*

My fellowship with God helps me make decisions by spiritual wisdom ~

> *1 Corinthians 2:6-16 However, we speak wisdom among those who are mature, yet not the wisdom of this age, nor of the rulers of this age, who are coming to nothing. 7 But we speak the wisdom of God in a mystery, the hidden wisdom which God ordained before the ages for our glory, 8 which none*

*of the rulers of this age knew; for had they known,
they would not have crucified the Lord of glory. 9
But as it is written: "Eye has not seen, nor ear
heard, Nor have entered into the heart of man The
things which God has prepared for those who love
Him." 10 But God has revealed them to us through
His Spirit. For the Spirit searches all things, yes, the
deep things of God. 11 For what man knows the
things of a man except the spirit of the man which is
in him? Even so no one knows the things of God
except the Spirit of God. 12 Now we have received,
not the spirit of the world, but the Spirit who is from
God, that we might know the things that have been
freely given to us by God. 13 These things we also
speak, not in words which man's wisdom teaches
but which the Holy Spirit teaches, comparing
spiritual things with spiritual. 14 But the natural
man does not receive the things of the Spirit of God,
for they are foolishness to him; nor can he know
them, because they are spiritually discerned. 15 But
he who is spiritual judges all things, yet he himself is
rightly judged by no one. 16 For "who has known the
mind of the Lord that he may instruct Him?" But we
have the mind of Christ. NKJV*

I bring every thought into captivity ~

*2 Corinthians 10:3-6 For though we walk in the
flesh, we do not war according to the flesh. 4 For the
weapons of our warfare are not carnal but mighty
in God for pulling down strongholds, 5 casting down
arguments and every high thing that exalts itself*

against the knowledge of God, bringing every thought into captivity to the obedience of Christ, 6 and being ready to punish all disobedience when your obedience is fulfilled. NKJV

I should please God with my thoughts ~

Philippians 4:8 Finally, brethren, whatever things are true, whatever things are noble, whatever things are just, whatever things are pure, whatever things are lovely, whatever things are of good report, if there is any virtue and if there is anything praiseworthy — meditate on these things. NKJV

I must guard my thoughts ~

Proverbs 4:23 Keep your heart with all diligence, For out of it spring the issues of life. NKJV

Sin wars against my mind ~

Romans 7:23 But I see another law in my members, warring against the law of my mind, and bringing me into captivity to the law of sin which is in my members. NKJV

I refuse to be double-minded ~

James 1:8 he is a double-minded man, unstable in all his ways. NKJV

Faith

I can do all things ~

> *Philippians 4:13 I can do all things through Christ who strengthens me. NKJV*

I believe despite what I see ~

> *Hebrews 11:1-2 Now faith is the substance of things hoped for, the evidence of things not seen. 2 For by it the elders obtained a good testimony. NKJV*

> *II Corinthians 5:7 For we walk by faith, not by sight. NKJV*

I do not doubt what God has said ~

> *James 1:5-6 If any of you lacks wisdom, let him ask of God, who gives to all liberally and without reproach, and it will be given to him. 6 But let him ask in faith, with no doubting, for he who doubts is like a wave of the sea driven and tossed by the wind. NKJV*

I abound in faith with thanksgiving ~

> *Colossians 2:6-7 As you therefore have received Christ Jesus the Lord, so walk in Him, 7 rooted and built up in Him and established in the faith, as you have been taught, abounding in it with thanksgiving. NKJV*

My faith is in Jesus ~

> *Galatians 2:20 I have been crucified with Christ; it is no longer I who live, but Christ lives in me; and the life which I now live in the flesh I live by faith in the Son of God, who loved me and gave Himself for me. NKJV*

I speak to my mountain ~

> *Mark 11:22-24 So Jesus answered and said to them, "Have faith in God. 23 For assuredly, I say to you, whoever says to this mountain, 'Be removed and be cast into the sea,' and does not doubt in his heart, but believes that those things he says will be done, he will have whatever he says. 24 Therefore I say to you, whatever things you ask when you pray, believe that you receive them, and you will have them. NKJV*

I read the Word to boost my faith ~

> *Romans 10:17 So then faith comes by hearing, and hearing by the word of God. NKJV*

I feed my faith and starve my doubts ~

> *Matthew 17:20-21 So Jesus said to them, "Because of your unbelief; for assuredly, I say to you, if you have faith as a mustard seed, you will say to this mountain, 'Move from here to there,' and it will move; and nothing will be impossible for you. 21 However, this kind does not go out except by prayer and fasting." NKJV*

My faith is more precious than gold ~

> *I Peter 1:7 that the genuineness of your faith, being much more precious than gold that perishes, though it is tested by fire, may be found to praise, honor, and glory at the revelation of Jesus Christ, NKJV*

My faith overcomes the world ~

> *I John 5:4 For whatever is born of God overcomes the world. And this is the victory that has overcome the world — our faith. NKJV*

I have faith and I speak to all obstacles in my way ~

> *Luke 17:5-6 And the apostles said to the Lord, "Increase our faith." 6 So the Lord said, "If you have faith as a mustard seed, you can say to this mulberry tree, 'Be pulled up by the roots and be planted in the sea,' and it would obey you. NKJV*

I quench all the fiery darts of the enemy with my shield of faith ~

> *Ephesians 6:16 above all, taking the shield of faith with which you will be able to quench all the fiery darts of the wicked one. NKJV*

Rejection

The Lord delivers me of all rejection ~

> *Psalms 34:17-20 The righteous cry out, and the Lord hears, And delivers them out of all their troubles. 18 The Lord is near to those who have a broken heart, And saves such as have a contrite spirit. 19 Many are the afflictions of the righteous, But the Lord delivers him out of them all. 20 He guards all his bones; Not one of them is broken. NKJV*

Though I am rejected by man I am precious to God ~

> *1 Peter 2:4 Coming to Him as to a living stone, rejected indeed by men, but chosen by God and precious, NKJV*

Jesus was rejected and overcame rejection on my behalf ~

> *John 15:18 "If the world hates you, you know that it hated Me before it hated you. NKJV*

Isaiah 53:3 He is despised and rejected by men, A Man of sorrows and acquainted with grief. And we hid, as it were, our faces from Him; He was despised, and we did not esteem Him. NKJV

Psalms 118:22 The stone which the builders rejected Has become the chief cornerstone. NKJV

I am sober and vigilant ~

1 Peter 5:8 Be sober, be vigilant; because your adversary the devil walks about like a roaring lion, seeking whom he may devour. NKJV

I cast my care on Him ~

1 Peter 5:7 casting all your care upon Him, for He cares for you. NKJV

Rejection is a doctrine of demons ~

1 Timothy 4:1 Now the Spirit expressly says that in latter times some will depart from the faith, giving heed to deceiving spirits and doctrines of demons, NKJV

God has not rejected me ~

Romans 8:15 For you did not receive the spirit of bondage again to fear, but you received the Spirit of adoption by whom we cry out, "Abba, Father." NKJV

**See our other books on Amazon.com

"Freedom From Endometriosis"

"Freedom From Migraines"

"Freedom From Acid Reflux"

"Freedom From High Blood Pressure"

"Freedom From Asthma"

"Freedom From Eczema"

"Freedom From Allergies"

"Freedom From Acne"

You can also purchase our books and other resources at

www.booksandgiftstogo.org and use promo code 20OFF code at checkout for a 20% discount!

Email me at poolofbethesdaschoolofhealing@gmail.com

with questions or testimonies.

---

ii Fear by Henry W. Wright pages 86-87

Made in the USA
Charleston, SC
25 January 2014